Copyright 2023

All right reserved. No part of this book should be reproduce without express permission of the author.

Reproduction of all or any part of this book is punishable under relevant law.

Table of Contents

PREVIEW
Eating nutritious foods that are high in calories is a good way to gain weight. It's also important to understand the reason why you're underweight.

Being underweight can be defined in a couple of ways. It can mean low weight for a person's height, defined as a body mass index (BMI) of less than 18.5. It also could be weight that is 15 to 20% below the typical weight for a person's age.

There are many reasons you may not be at your goal weight. Recovering from an illness or losing weight as you age are two examples. It's also common for athletes to want to gain weight as muscle.

It is best to see your health care provider if you lost weight unexpectedly. Your provider or a dietitian can help you gain weight in a healthy way. Together, you can create a plan based on your needs.

Weight gain, especially if it's new, can signal a number of health conditions. For example, someone with heart failure might experience weight gain from fluid retention—which might appear as swelling in the feet, ankles, legs, or belly. "This would likely be accompanied by symptoms such as fatigue or shortness of breath," Dr. Apovian says.

Other underlying conditions associated with weight gain include

Diabetes

Certain kidney diseases

Sleep apnea (pauses in breathing during sleep)

Thyroid problems.

Gaining weight can be difficult for some people. With a few changes, you can gradually reach a healthy weight.

Being underweight could mean you're missing out on vitamins and minerals.

This could lead to health problems such as a weak immune system and bone fractures.

WEIGH GAIN DIET RECIPES

BREAKFAST
1. Burrito Wrap with Bacon and Avocado
Prep Time: 10 Minutes

Cook Time: 15 Minutes

Servings: 2

Ingredients

- 2 eggs
- 2 tablespoon heavy cream (optional)
- To taste salt
- To taste pepper
- 2 teaspoon butter
- 2 tablespoon mayonnaise
- 1 cup romaine lettuce (chopped)
- 1 roma tomato (sliced)
- 4 cooked bacon strips
- ½ avocado (sliced)

Instructions

1. Whisk the eggs well with the heavy cream, salt and pepper.
2. Heat up a non-stick pan to a medium heat.
3. Melt half the butter in the pan, and pour in half the egg mixture. Immediately tilt the pan back and forth to ensure the egg covers the entire base.
4. Cover the pan and let the cook for about a minute.

5. When you are able to move the entire crepe when shaking the pan back and forth, carefully flip it over with a spatula.
6. When it's fully cooked, transfer to a paper towel to remove excess oiliness.
7. Repeat with the other half of the egg mix.
8. Spread the mayonaisse on the crepe.
9. Add the lettuce, tomato, bacon and avocado.
10. Season with salt and pepper.
11. Roll and enjoy!

2. Egg Muffins with Mushrooms and Spinach
Prep Time: 20 Minutes

Cook Time: 25 Minutes

Servings: 12

Ingredients

- 1 tablespoon olive oil
- Salt
- 6 oz mushrooms, thinly sliced
- 6 eggs
- ¼ cup milk
- ¼ teaspoon salt
- 2 cups cheddar cheese, shredded
- ¾ cup spinach, cooked and drained (about 8 oz fresh spinach)

Instructions

1. In a large skillet, heat olive oil on medium-high heat, and add thinly sliced mushrooms, sprinkle with salt, and cook for about 10 minutes until mushrooms soften and release juices.
2. Preheat oven to 350 degrees. Use a regular 12-cup muffin pan. Spray the muffin pan with non-stick cooking spray.
3. In a large bowl, beat eggs until smooth. Add milk, salt, Cheddar cheese and mix. Stir spinach, cooked mushrooms into the egg mixture. Ladle the egg mixture into greased muffin cups ¾ full.

4. Bake for 25 minutes. Remove from the oven, let the muffins cool for 30 minutes before removing them from the pan.

3. Italian Casserole
Prep Time: 10 Minutes

Cook Time: 55 Minutes

Servings: 10

Ingredients

- 1 butternut squash long part only, peeled and sliced into 1/4" rounds
- 1 Tbsp coconut oil for greasing baking dish and squash, sea salt for roasting
- 1 Tbsp coconut oil for cooking sausage and veggies
- 1 lb pork sausage casings removed if necessary, no added sugar
- 1 red bell pepper diced
- 1 onion medium, diced
- 3 cloves garlic minced
- Pinch crushed red pepper
- 3 oz sun dried tomatoes (Whole30 compliant) chopped, (about 3/4 cup packed), soften first by soaking if too hard
- 2 tsp Italian seasoning blend
- 12 large eggs
- 1/2 cup coconut milk full fat
- 1/2 tsp fine grain sea salt
- 1/8 tsp black pepper
- 3 Tbsp nutritional yeast optional, for flavor
- Parsley minced, for garnish

Instructions

1. Preheat your oven to 425 F and grease a 9x13"
   casserole dish with coconut oil.
2. Toss the butternut squash rounds with coconut oil
   and sea salt to taste (generous pinch for me) and
   arrange, (overlapping since they will shrink after
   roasting) over the bottom of your casserole dish, and
   along the sides if desired.
3. Place the casserole dish with the butternut in the
   preheated oven and roast until softened - overcooking
   will lead to mushy squash.
4. Meanwhile, heat a large skillet over med heat, add a
   tsp of coconut oil, crumble sausage into skillet, and
   sprinkle with crushed red pepper. Cook, breaking up
   lumps, until browned, then remove to a plate and set
   aside.
5. Add another tsp coconut oil to skillet, then add the
   peppers and onions. Cook until just softened, then
   add the garlic and cook another 30 seconds.
6. Once garlic is soft, add sun dried tomatoes and cooked
   sausage to heat through, then remove skillet from
   heat.
7. In a large bowl or measuring cup, whisk together the
   eggs, coconut milk, Italian seasoning, salt, pepper,
   and nutritional yeast (if using), until very smooth.
8. To assemble casserole, arrange the sausage veggie
   mixture over the cooked butternut crust, leaving
   excess grease/water in the skillet.
9. Pour the egg mixture over the top evenly, then bake in
   the preheated oven for 22-25 minutes or until egg
   mixture is set in the center and begins to puff up.
   Don't allow it to overcook or turn brown!
10. Garnish with parsley or other fresh herbs before
    serving. Allow casserole to sit for 10 minutes before

slicing and serving. You can also refrigerate or freeze to reheat at a later point. Enjoy!

4. Sloppy Joe Sweet Potato
Prep Time: 10 Minutes

Cook Time: 30 Minutes

Servings: 4

Ingredients

- 2 sweet potatoes (cut into bite-sized cubes)
- 1 lb ground beef (500g)
- 1 green pepper (diced)
- 1 onion (diced)
- 1 tomato (diced)
- 1 garlic clove (minced)
- 3 tablespoon Worcestershire sauce
- 3 tablespoon ketchup
- 1 tablespoon spicy mustard
- ½ cup water
- To taste salt and pepper
- To taste butter
- 4 eggs

Instructions

1. Put the sweet potato in a small pot and cover with cold water. Place on the stove over a high heat and bring to a boil. Cook for about 10 minutes, or until soft. Strain water and set aside.
2. While the sweet potato boils: Brown the ground beef in a sauté pan, together with the onion, green pepper and tomato.

3. Add the garlic, worcestershire sauce, ketchup, mustard, water, salt and pepper. Cover and simmer uncovered until thickened, about 20-25 minutes.
4. Optional: When the sweet potato is done, sear the cubes in a piping hot pan with some butter and season with salt and pepper.
5. Top the sweet potato with the sloppy joe and an egg fried to your liking.

5. Bacon Cauliflower Skillet
Prep Time: 10 Minutes

Cook Time: 15 Minutes

Servings: 2

Ingredients

- 2 cups cauliflower [chopped fine in food processor]
- ½ brown onion [diced]
- ½ red bell pepper [diced]
- 4 bacon strips [cut into bite-sized pieces]
- 4 eggs [boiled to your preferences. we boiled ours for 8 minutes to medium hard]
- ½ cup heavy cream
- ½ teaspoon paprika
- 1 tablespoon butter
- To taste salt and pepper

Instructions

1. Sauté the bacon and onion together until the bacon is cooked and the onion is soft.
2. Add the cauliflower, red bell pepper, paprika, butter and season with salt and pepper.
3. Sauté everything together until the cauliflower is cooked to your liking [about 5-10 minutes]
4. Add the heavy cream and stir until everything is hot and blended.
5. Add the boiled eggs on top and garnish with fresh parsley.
6. Serve hot and enjoy!

6. Smoked Salmon Bowl
Prep Time: 5 Minutes

Cook Time: 20 Minutes

Servings: 2

Ingredients

- 4 eggs
- 2 tablespoon whole milk
- To taste salt and pepper
- 1 tablespoon butter
- ½ avocado [sliced]
- 8 small vine tomatoes [oven roasted @ 350°F/180°C for 20 minutes or cheat and set it under the broiler for a couple of minutes]
- To taste smoked salmon
- 1 tablespoon fresh chopped chives
- 2 tablespoon creme fraiche

Instructions

1. Whisk the eggs with the whole milk, salt and pepper.
2. Melt the butter over a medium heat and cook the eggs until they are done, but still moist.
3. Serve the eggs right away with the vine tomatoes, avocado and a couple ribbons of smoked salmon.
4. Add a dollop of creme fraiche to each plate and top everything with fresh chopped chives.

7. Low-Carb Sweet Potato with Poached Egg
Prep Time: 10 Minutes

Cook Time: 10 Minutes

Servings: 4

Ingredients

- 2 sweet potato (peeled and shredded - should yield about 4 cups)
- 4 eggs
- 8 bacon strips (cooked crispy and roughly chopped)
- To taste salt and pepper
- ½ cup fresh basil (roughl chopped)
- 1 tbsp oil (own preference)

Instructions

1. Cook the sweet potato in the oil over medium-high heat for approximately 10 minutes, until cooked. Season with salt and pepper to taste.
2. While the sweet potato cooks, bring a shallow sauce pan filled with water to the boil. Once boiling, bring down to a light simmer. Crack the eggs into the simmering water and let cook for 2-3 minutes for a soft egg. Remove with a slotted spoon.
3. Divide the sweet potato hash into plates, top each with an egg, chopped bacon and fresh basil.

8. Keto Chicken Bake

Prep Time: 10 Minutes

Cook Time: 20 Minutes

Servings: 2

Ingredients

- ½ lb chicken breast (250g) (cut into bite-sized chunks)
- ½ red bell pepper (roughly chopped)
- 1 onion (sliced)
- 2 eggs
- 1 fresh jalapeño pepper (seeded and diced)
- ½ cup cheese (shredded)
- To taste salt and pepper
- 1 tablespoon oil (for cooking)

Instructions

1. Preheat the oven 350°F/180°C.
2. Sauté the onion, bell peppers and jalapeño pepper in a little bit of oil for about 5 minutes. Season with salt and pepper.
3. Transfer to an oven safe dish.
4. Add the chicken to the dish. (We used leftover chicken.
5. Crack the eggs into the dish and sprinkle the cheese on top.
6. Slide into the oven for approximately 15-20 minutes.

9. Veggie Stack
Prep Time: 10 Minutes

Cook Time: 20 Minutes

Servings: 2

Ingredients

- 2 large portobello mushrooms
- 1 medium zucchini [cut in half and sliced thinly]
- 1 red bell pepper [julienne]
- 1 cup baby spinach
- 2 tablespoon crumbled feta cheese
- ¼ cup mayonnaise
- 1 teaspoon dried dill
- To taste salt and pepper

Instructions

Preheat oven 350°F.

1. Sprinkle the mushrooms with salt and pepper and bake for 20 minutes.
2. While that cooks, sauté the zucchini in a little bit of butter and set aside.
3. Then, sauté the bell peppers and set aside.
4. Once the mushrooms are ready, slide onto plates and top with spinach, zucchini and the red bell pepper.
5. Add some dill mayo and top with the feta cheese.

10. Coconut Flour Pancakes
Prep Time: 5 Minutes

Cook Time: 15 Minutes

Servings: 4

Ingredients

- 4 eggs
- 3 tablespoon coconut flour
- 2 teaspoon vanilla essence
- 2 teaspoon baking powder
- 1 tablespoon honey (or use any diet compliant liquid sweetener)

Instructions

1. Mix all ingredients together until smooth and lump free.
2. Melt a small amount of butter in a nonstick pan over a medium heat.
3. Add 3-4 scoops of batter into the pan depending on the size of the pan.
4. Cook for 1-2 minutes per side. They're usually ready to flip when small bubbles form on the surface of the pancakes.
5. Serve while hot!

LUNCH
11. Eggs in Purgatory
Prep Time: 5 Minutes

Cook Time: 20 Minutes

Servings: 4

Ingredients

- 1 can diced tomato
- 6 eggs
- 2 tablespoon butter
- ½ tablespoon minced garlic
- 1 teaspoon dried oregano
- 1 teaspoon dried basil
- 2 tablespoon parmesan
- To taste salt and pepper

Instructions

1. Melt the butter in a large skillet over a medium high heat.
2. Add the garlic and spices and saute until aromatic.
3. Add the canned tomato, salt and pepper. Bring to a boil.
4. Lower the temperature to a simmer and cook for about 10-15 minutes.
5. Now, use a spoon to create 6 evenly spaced dents in the tomato sauce and crack the eggs into each dents.
6. Cover and cook for 4-6 minutes.
7. Top with shredded parmesan and serve immediately.

12. Chimichurri Sauce
Prep Time: 3 Minutes

Cook Time: 2 Minutes

Servings: 10

Ingredients

- 2 cups fresh parsley
- 1 cup fresh cilantro
- 4 cloves garlic
- 2 teaspoon dried oregano
- 1 teaspoon red chili flakes
- ¼ shallots (roughly chopped)
- ¼ cup lemon juice
- ¼ cup red wine vinegar
- 1 cup avocado oil (or oil of preference)
- To taste salt and pepper

Instructions

1. Blits everything together in a food processor to desired consistency, but leaving it on the chunkier side is preferable.

13. Keto Guacamole
Prep Time: 10 Minutes

Cook Time: 00 Minutes

Servings: 6

Ingredients

- 2 avocado (sliced into cubes)
- ¼ cup red onion (finely diced)
- 1 roma tomato (cut the tomato into quarters, remove the seeds removed and then chop into small cubes)
- ½ lime (just the juice)
- ½ cup fresh cilantro (roughly chopped)
- 1 teaspoon minced garlic
- 1 pickled jalapeño pepper (optional) (finely chopped)
- To taste salt and pepper

Instructions

2. Chuck everything into a bowl and mash it up to your desired level of chunkiness.
3. Tips and Tricks:
4. When storing the guacamole, press the guacamole down into a bowl and press plastic wrap down on the surface of the guacamole to limit air exposure as much as possible.

14. Butternut Squash, Kale & Ground Beef Bowl
Prep Time: 00 Minutes

Cook Time: 2 Minutes

Servings: 1

Ingredients

- ½ small onion, finely diced
- 1-2 button mushrooms, chopped
- 150 g lean ground grass fed beef
- Salt and pepper to taste
- 5 kale leaves, stems removed and chopped (you can sub collard or baby spinach)
- ¼ large butternut squash, cooked and cooled (that's about 1½ cup)
- ¼ cup full fat coconut milk
- 1 tsp garam masala
- ½ tsp spicy curry
- ¼ tsp ground ginger
- ¼ tsp ground cinnamon
- 1-2 tbsp organic toasted coconut shavings
- 1-2 tbsp full fat coconut milk

Instructions

1. In a heavy skillet set over medium high heat melt a little bit of coconut oil. When oil is nice and hot, add onions, mushrooms, salt and pepper and cook until the veggies are fragrant and softened, about 2-3 minutes.

2. Add ground beef, garam masala, curry, ginger and cinnamon and continue cooking until the beef is no longer pink in color.
3. Throw in the chopped kale and cook, stirring delicately, until the kale starts to wilt and turns a vivid dark green.
4. Stir in cooked squash and coconut milk and stir to break down the squash and incorporate the coconut milk. Continue cooking just until heated through.
5. Transfer to a bowl (its very important that you use a bowl here, else you would totally lose the right to call this a breakfast bowl) and garnish with a handful of toasted coconut and a few tablespoons of thick and delicious coconut milk.

15. 4 Minute Microwave Butternut Squash Chips

Prep Time: 15 Minutes

Cook Time: 4 Minutes

Servings: 2

Ingredients

- 1 butternut squash (peeled and sliced thinly with a mandolin)
- 2 tablespoon avocado oil (or any oil of preference)
- To taste salt/seasoning of choice

Instructions

1. Toss the sliced butternut, oil and seasoning together in a bowl.
2. Arrange the slices in a single on a microwaveable plate.
3. Microwave for approximately 4 minutes per batch.

Tips and Tricks:

1. The chips are ready when they start to darken in color. They'll crisp up once they are cooled down. If they're chewy, not crispy, they need to cook longer so adjust the time for the next batch.
2. One whole butternut takes 3-4 batches, depending on the size of the plate you use to cook them in the microwave.

16. Butternut Squash, Kale & Ground Beef Bowl
Prep Time: 2 Minutes

Cook Time: 3 Minutes

Servings: 1

Ingredients

- ½ small onion, finely diced
- 1-2 button mushrooms, chopped
- 150 g lean ground grass fed beef
- Salt and pepper to taste
- 5 kale leaves, stems removed and chopped (you can sub collard or baby spinach)
- ¼ large butternut squash, cooked and cooled (that's about 1½ cup)
- ¼ cup full fat coconut milk
- 1 tsp garam masala
- ½ tsp spicy curry
- ¼ tsp ground ginger
- ¼ tsp ground cinnamon
- 1-2 tbsp organic toasted coconut shavings
- 1-2 tbsp full fat coconut milk

Instructions

1. In a heavy skillet set over medium high heat melt a little bit of coconut oil. When oil is nice and hot, add onions, mushrooms, salt and pepper and cook until the veggies are fragrant and softened, about 2-3 minutes.

2. Add ground beef, garam masala, curry, ginger and cinnamon and continue cooking until the beef is no longer pink in color.
3. Throw in the chopped kale and cook, stirring delicately, until the kale starts to wilt and turns a vivid dark green.
4. Stir in cooked squash and coconut milk and stir to break down the squash and incorporate the coconut milk. Continue cooking just until heated through.
5. Transfer to a bowl (its very important that you use a bowl here, else you would totally lose the right to call this a breakfast bowl) and garnish with a handful of toasted coconut and a few tablespoons of thick and delicious coconut milk.

17. Keto Guacamole
Prep Time: 10 Minutes

Cook Time: 00 Minutes

Servings: 6

Ingredients

- 2 avocado (sliced into cubes)
- ¼ cup red onion (finely diced)
- 1 roma tomato (cut the tomato into quarters, remove the seeds removed and then chop into small cubes)
- ½ lime (just the juice)
- ½ cup fresh cilantro (roughly chopped)
- 1 teaspoon minced garlic
- 1 pickled jalapeño pepper (optional) (finely chopped)
- to taste salt and pepper

Instructions

1. Chuck everything into a bowl and mash it up to your desired level of chunkiness.

Tips and Tricks:

2. When storing the guacamole, press the guacamole down into a bowl and press plastic wrap down on the surface of the guacamole to limit air exposure as much as possible.

18. One Pot Paleo Chicken
Prep Time: 15 Minutes

Cook Time: 30 Minutes

Servings: 6

Ingredients

- 1 lb chicken pieces (500g)
- 1 yellow onion (diced)
- 2 cups zucchini (350g) (cut into rounds)
- 2 cups baby potatoes (sliced in half)
- 2 cups carrots (peeled and sliced into rounds)
- 2 cups white button mushrooms (250g) (sliced half)
- 2 cups hot water

Herbs and Spices:

- 1 teaspoon dried thyme
- 1 teaspoon ground coriander
- 1 tablespoon salt (use 2 teaspoon if you're using fine table salt)
- ½ teaspoon black pepper

Instructions

3. Heat up a large pot and sear the chicken, skin side down. It needs to get a GOOD sear, so don't be scared to let it sit for a while.
4. Now, add all the rest of the ingredients and bring to a boil.
5. Lower the heat so it doesn't boil too vigorously.
6. Put a lid on the pot and let it boil for 30 minutes.

7. When done, I like to separate the vegetables, chicken
    and sauce.
8. Garnish with freshly chopped parsley and serve
    immediately.

Tips and Tricks:

1. If the sauce is too runny - remove the chicken and
    vegetable and let it simmer for a few minutes longer in
    order to reduce and thicken.
2. You can also add a knob of cold butter from the fridge
    to help thicken the sauce once you've removed it from
    the stove.

19. Keto Meatloaf

Prep Time: 10 Minutes

Cook Time: 45 Minutes

Servings: 8

Ingredients

For the Meatloaf Stuffing

- 2 lb ground beef (1kg)
- 4 eggs
- 2 onions (medium sized) (Finely chopped)
- 2 celery stalks (Finely chopped)
- ½ cup shredded cheese (We prefer Gouda or medium cheddar)
- ½ cup parmesan cheese
- ½ cup almond flour
- 2 tablespoon minced garlic
- 2 tablespoon olive oil
- 2 tablespoon coconut aminos (Can use soy sauce as well)
- 2 teaspoon dried oregano
- 1 teaspoon chili powder (Mexican mild chili powder)
- 3 teaspoon salt (We use coarse salt, so use less if you're using fine table salt)
- 1 teaspoon ground black pepper
- ½ cup ketchup

Instructions

Pre-heat the oven to 400F/200C

1. Add all the ingredients for the meatloaf in a large
   mixing bowl - mix until well combined. Use your
   hands to make it easier.
2. On a lined baking sheet, form the ground beef mixture
   into loaf shape.
3. Spread the ketchup over the top of the meatloaf. Use
   more if required.
4. Slide into the oven and cook for 35-45 minutes.
   Cooking time will depend on the exact
   shape/thickness of your meatloaf. Its cooked when it
   reaches an internal temperature of 160F/70C.

Tips and Tricks:

1. Be sure to use ketchup compliant to your personal
   diet requirements. For low-carb, keto, paleo and
   whole 30 approved ketchup - we use our own personal
   recipe. Find it here.

20. Stuffed Bell Peppers without Rice (Keto Friendly)
Prep Time: 10 Minutes

Cook Time: 45 Minutes

Servings: 6

Ingredients

For the Meatloaf Stuffing

- 1 lb ground beef (500g)
- 2 eggs
- 1 medium onion (Finely chopped)
- 2 celery stalks
- ½ cup shredded cheese (We prefer Gouda or medium cheddar)
- ¼ cup parmesan cheese
- ¼ cup almond flour
- 1 tablespoon minced garlic
- 1 tablespoon olive oil
- 1 tablespoon coconut aminos (Can use soy sauce as well)
- 1 teaspoon dried oregano
- 1 teaspoon chili powder (Mexican mild chili powder)
- 2 teaspoon salt (We use coarse salt, so use less if you're using fine table salt)
- ½ teaspoon ground black pepper

For the rest:

- 4 bell peppers (Sliced in half, ribs and seeds removed)
- 8 bacon strips
- 1 cup ketchup

Instructions

Turn on the oven to 400F/200C

2. Mix all the ingredients for the ground beef in a large mixing bowl. Set aside.
3. Wash the bell peppers and then slice them in half. Use a spoon to carefully scrape out the ribs and seeds. Remove the entire stem area of the top half as well.
4. Spread approximately 1 tablespoon of ketchup on the inside of each pepper.
5. Add 2 strips of bacon to each pepper.
6. Divide the beef stuffing evenly between the peppers.
7. Fold the bacon over top of the ground beef.
8. Spread approximately 1 tablespoon on ketchup over the top of the bacon and ground beef.
9. Put the peppers into a sheet pan or oven dish and slide into the oven for 45 minutes.
10. The stuffed peppers are done when they reach an internal temperature of 160F/70C.

Tips and Tricks:

1. The bacon strips are completely optional and the recipe works perfectly fine without it - it does add an extra layer of yumminess though.
2. Be sure to use ketchup compliant to your personal diet requirements. For low-carb, keto, paleo and whole 30 approved ketchup - we use our own personal recipe. Find it here.

DINNER
21. Crustless Cheesy Chicken and Asparagus Pie
Prep Time: 15 Minutes

Cook Time: 45 Minutes

Servings: 4

Ingredients

- ½ lb cooked chicken [250g, about 2 chicken breasts shredded with two forks]
- 2 white onions [chopped]
- 1 can asparagus [14oz/400g can size - drained and chopped into bitesize pieces]
- 1 cup shredded cheddar cheese
- 1 teaspoon paprika
- ½ teaspoon mustard powder
- ½ teaspoon garlic powder
- 1 teaspoon salt [we used regular fine table salt]
- ½ teaspoon white pepper
- Pinch cayenne pepper
- ½ cup milk
- 4 large eggs
- 1 tablespoon oil [of choice, for cooking and greasing your pie dish]

Instructions

Preheat the oven to 350F/180C

1. Cook the onion in a little bit of oil until the start to brown, 10-15 minutes. Use the time while the onion

cooks to prepare the rest of the ingredients, but remember to stir the onions every minute or so.

2. Once the onions are nicely browned, add the chicken and all the spices into the pan and stir until everything is well combined
3. Use a paper towel to wipe a bit of oil on the inside of your pie dish.
4. Now, add the onion and chicken to the pie dish.
5. Add the asparagus pieces of top and gently mix.
6. Top with the shredded cheese.
7. Now, in a small bowl, mix together the milk and eggs and carefully pour over the ingredients in the pie dish. Be sure to gently shake the dish a little bit to help the egg mix spread into all the nooks and crannies.
8. Slide into the oven and bake for 45 minutes.
9. When done, allow to stand for 5-10 minutes before serving.

Tips and Tricks:

1. This is a great recipe for leftover or rotisserie chicken, but if you don't have leftover chicken you can lightly season two butterflied chicken breasts with salt and pepper and allow it to cook in a second pan while you brown the onions and prep/measure the rest of the ingredients.
2. I used a 10" pie dish.
3. This recipe is also great the next day and can be eaten cold for a refreshing lunch!

22. Healthy Chicken Nuggets
Prep Time: 15 Minutes

Cook Time: 15 Minutes

Servings: 4

Ingredients

- 1 lb ground chicken (can also lightly blend chicken breasts) (500g)
- For The Crumb Coating:
- ½ cup breadcrumbs (we use our crumbs made from our homemade sourdough bread)
- ½ cup parmesan cheese (this recipe will also work fine using only parmesan cheese, just sub the breadcrumbs for more cheese)
- 1 teaspoon onion flakes (can use ½ teaspoon onion powder)
- 1 teaspoon garlic powder
- 1 teaspoon paprika
- 1 teaspoon dried thyme
- 1 teaspoon salt
- ½ teaspoon pepper

For The Egg Wash

- 1 eggs
- 2 tablespoon milk

Instructions

Preheat the oven to 425F/200C.

1. Prepare a baking sheet with baking paper.
2. Mix all the ingredients for the crumb coating in a shallow dish.
3. Mix the ingredients for the egg wash into a seperate shallow dish.
4. With the chicken, about 2-3 tablespoon worth at a time, form nugget shapes.
5. Dip the nugget into the egg wash until coated.
6. Transfer to the crumb mix and coat evenly.
7. Arrange on the baking sheet.
8. Once you've finished all the chicken, slide the tray into the preheated oven for approximately 15 minutes, turning once halfway.
9. Serve while warm!

23. Keto French Onion Soup
Prep Time: 30 Minutes

Cook Time: 2hrs 2 Minutes

Servings: 8

Ingredients

- 2 lb stewing beef (1kg) (cut into smaller chunks)
- 6 yellow onions (thinly sliced)
- 2 red onions (thinly sliced)
- 4 tablespoon olive oil
- 2 tablespoon butter
- 1 teaspoon dried rosemary
- 1 teaspoon celery salt
- 1 teaspoon dried thyme
- ½ teaspoon ground black pepper
- 8 cups water
- ½ cup apple juice (you can substitute the apple juice and apple cider vinegar for ½ cup white wine)
- 1 tablespoon apple cider vinegar
- To taste salt
- To taste shredded cheese optional (swiss or mozarella, for topping)

Instructions

1. In a large pot, high heat - sear the chunks of stewing beef in a little bit of oil, and then set aside. Lower temperature to medium.
2. In the same pot add the rest of the oil, butter and all the sliced onions. Cook on a medium until carmelized,

this can take 20+ minutes. You want to spend a lot of time on this step to get good flavor out of the onions.

3. Once the onions are carmelized, return beef to the pot. Add the garlic and spices and allow to cook together for a minute or two.
4. Now add the apple juice and apple cider vinegar (or white wine) and cook for another minute or two.
5. Now add the water, allow it to come to a boil, and then lower the heat so it can simmer for anywhere from 1-2 hours depending on the beef.
6. Once the beef is tender and can easily shred apart, the soup is done.
7. Remove the beef and save for another meal, shred it up and return to the soup for something more hearty and filling, or shred the beef and make french dip sandwiches to dip into the soup.
8. If you're doing regular french onion soup, ladle the soup into soup bowl and add a nice helping of shredded cheese on top.

24. Ground Beef and Broccoli
Prep Time: 10 Minutes

Cook Time: 20 Minutes

Servings: 6

Ingredients

- 1 lb ground beef (500g)
- 5 cups broccoli florets
- 3 cups cauliflower rice
- 1 onion (thinly sliced)
- 2 tablespoon ghee (or coconut oil for cooking)

Sauce:

- 6 tablespoon soy sauce (or coconut aminos)
- ½ teaspoon black pepper
- 2 teaspoon sesame seeds
- 2 tablespoon raw honey
- 1 tablespoon minced garlic
- 1 teaspoon grated ginger
- ¼ cup water (optional)

Instructions

1. Add all the ingredients for the sauce (except the water) into a small bowl and mix. Set aside.
2. Add the onion and ground beef to a large skillet with the ghee and sauté until the beef is browned. 5-10 minutes.

3. Add the broccoli, cauliflower and sauce and cook until
   the broccoli reached your desired level of tenderness.
   5-10 minutes.
4. Garnish with freshly chopped cilantro, red pepper
   flakes and more sesame seeds. (Optional)
5. Serve and enjoy!

25. Instant Pot Ground Beef Hamburger Soup
Prep Time: 15 Minutes

Cook Time: 12 Minutes

Servings: 6

Ingredients

- 1lb ground beef [500g]
- 2 large onions (diced)
- 2 large carrots (sliced)
- 2 cups baby potatoes (halved, cubed if using sweet potato)
- 2 cups green beans (sliced)
- 1 tablespoon minced garlic
- 4 cups beef broth/stock
- 2 canned tomato
- 2 tablespoon dijon mustard
- 2 teaspoon salt
- 2 teaspoon dried oregano
- 2 teaspoon dried thyme
- 2 teaspoon chili powder
- 1 teaspoon parsley

Instructions

1. Set the Instant Pot to the Sauté setting and sauté the ground beef and onion until the ground beef in browned.
2. Add all the rest of the ingredients to the pot and stir.
3. Seal the instant pot and use the manual setting - High Pressure and 12 Minutes on the timer.

4. Use quick or natural release.
5. Serve and enjoy!

Tips and Tricks:

1. Omit the potato, or substitute it with cauliflower (or any other vegetable of your own choice) to make this hamburger soup recipe low carb and keto approved.

26. Chimichurri Steak
Prep Time: 5 Minutes

Cook Time: 8 Minutes

Servings: 6

Ingredients

- 1 steak (we used a large 50oz steak, about ½" thick)
- ½ cup chimichurri sauce (add more or less to taste)
- To taste salt and pepper
- 2 teaspoon ground coriande (optional)
- 2 teaspoon dried thyme (optional)

Instructions

2. Allow the steak to come to room temperature. Take it out of the fridge about 20-30 minutes before you're ready to cook it.
3. Season the steak generously with salt and pepper. Don't be shy on the salt - its pretty hard to over salt a steak. Add any other seasonings or herbs at this point if you'd like.
4. Cook the steak about 3-4 minutes per side. (This is assuming you have a ½" thick steak. Check the post for a link on how to cook the perfect steak).
5. Cover the steak with foil and allow to rest for 10 minutes.
6. Slice into strips and top with chimichurri sauce to taste.
7. Enjoy!

27. Homemade Spaghetti Sauce
Prep Time: 10 Minutes

Cook Time: 30 Minutes

Servings: 8

Ingredients

- 1 lb ground beef (500g)
- 2 onions (diced)
- 2 cans diced tomatoes (14oz cans)
- 2 carrots (peeled and grated)
- 2 garlic cloves (minced)
- 1 cup beef broth
- 2 tablespoon tomato paste
- ½ teaspoon celery seeds
- 2 teaspoon dried oregano
- ¼ teaspoon red chili flakes
- To taste salt and ground black pepper
- Garnish freshly chopped parsley (optional)

Instructions

1. Sauté the onions, ground beef and garlic together until the beef is browned in a pot.
2. Add everything else and stir. Be sure to season well with salt and pepper.
3. Cover and allow to simmer for 25-30 minutes.
4. Serve and enjoy!

28. Keto Guacamole
Prep Time: 10 Minutes

Cook Time: 10 Minutes

Servings: 6

Ingredients

- 2 avocado (sliced into cubes)
- ¼ cup red onion (finely diced)
- 1 roma tomato (cut the tomato into quarters, remove the seeds removed and then chop into small cubes)
- ½ lime (just the juice)
- ½ cup fresh cilantro (roughly chopped)
- 1 teaspoon minced garlic
- 1 pickled jalapeño pepper (optional) (finely chopped)
- To taste salt and pepper

Instructions

1. Chuck everything into a bowl and mash it up to your desired level of chunkiness.

Tips and Tricks:

2. When storing the guacamole, press the guacamole down into a bowl and press plastic wrap down on the surface of the guacamole to limit air exposure as much as possible.

29. Keto Philly Cheesesteak Casserole (with Ground Beef)
Prep Time: 15 Minutes

Cook Time: 25 Minutes

Servings: 6

Ingredients

- 500 g ground beef (1lb)
- 2 bell peppers (diced) (we used one yellow and one green)
- 1 yellow onion (diced)
- 250 g white mushrooms (approximately 8oz - sliced)
- 1 tablespoon minced garlic
- 4 large eggs
- ¼ cup heavy cream
- 1 cup cheddar cheese (grated)
- Herbs and Spices
- 2 teaspoon paprika
- 1 teaspoon mexican chili powder
- 2 teaspoon dried thyme
- 2 teaspoon dried basil
- 2 teaspoon salt (add more or less to taste)

Instructions

Preheat the oven to 200°C/400°F

3. In a pan, sauté the onions, mushrooms and diced green pepper together until the onions are translucent.

4. Transfer to a casserole dish. (I used a 30cm X 20cm or 8"x6" dish)
5. In the same pan add the ground beef, garlic, herbs and spices. Brown the ground beef until just barely cooked, and slightly pink.
6. Transfer to the casserole dish.
7. Mix everything together well.
8. In a small bowl, mix the eggs and cream together and pour over the beef and vegetables.
9. Top with cheese and slide into the oven for about 25 minutes. Until the cheese is golden and bubbly.

Tips and Tricks:

1. We always serve this with a dollop of our yummy Homemade Mayonnaise.
2. We like serving this casserole by offering a variety of toppings with it for everyone to pick and choose according to their own taste. Here's what we like:
1. Shredded Lettuce
2. Chopped Tomato
3. Pickles
4. Sliced Olives
5. Banana Peppers

30. The Best Easy Low Carb Keto Green Bean Casserole
Prep Time: 10 Minutes

Cook Time: 20 Minutes

Servings: 6

Ingredients

- 3 cups fresh green beans (sliced into smaller pieces)
- 2/5 cups button mushrooms (sliced)
- 2 onions (sliced)
- 1 garlic cloves (minced)
- ½ cup cream cheese
- ½ cup chicken stock
- ½ cup cheddar (grated)
- ¼ teaspoon nutmeg
- To taste salt and ground black pepper

Instructions

Preheat the oven to 200°C/400°F

1. Boil the green beans in well salted water until fork tender. Approximately 10 minutes. Drain the water and set aside. (Important: The water for boiling the green beans should be WELL salted - think sea water salty).
2. While the green beans boil, sauté the onions, mushrooms and garlic until caramelized. Season with salt, pepper and the nutmeg.
3. Add the chicken stock and be sure to scrape all the bits from the bottom of the pan.

4. Add the cream cheese and allow to melt and warm up. Taste test and add salt if needed.
5. Mix in the green beans until everything is evenly combined and transfer everything into a casserole dish.
6. Top with cheddar and pop into the oven until the cheese is melted and bubble. About 10 minutes.

Tips and Tricks:

1. For an optional, but delicious topping: Set aside a small handful of your sliced onions and lightly coat them in coconut flour. Add oil to a small pan and fry the onions until golden. Let them sit on a paper towel when you remove them from the oil and lightly salt.
2. Sprinkle these on top of the casserole before serving.

www.ingramcontent.com/pod-product-compliance
Lightning Source LLC
Chambersburg PA
CBHW071126260726
48661CB00006B/2706